LABORATORY MANUAL AND WORKBOOK FOR
FUCHS'S PRINCIPLES OF RADIOGRAPHIC EXPOSURE, PROCESSING AND QUALITY CONTROL, Third Edition

LABORATORY MANUAL AND WORKBOOK
FOR
FUCHS'S PRINCIPLES OF RADIOGRAPHIC EXPOSURE, PROCESSING AND QUALITY CONTROL, Third Edition

By

QUINN B. CARROLL, M.Ed., R.T.

Director, Medical Radiography Department
Laramie County Community College
Cheyenne, Wyoming

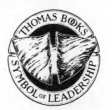

CHARLES C THOMAS • PUBLISHER
Springfield • Illinois • U.S.A.

Published and Distributed Throughout the World by
CHARLES C THOMAS • PUBLISHER
2600 South First Street
Springfield, Illinois 62717

© *1985 by* CHARLES C THOMAS • PUBLISHER
ISBN 0-398-05082-1

With THOMAS BOOKS *careful attention is given to all details of manufacturing and
design. It is the Publisher's desire to present books that are satisfactory as to their physical
qualities and artistic possibilities and appropriate for their particular use.* THOMAS
BOOKS *will be true to those laws of quality that assure a good name and good will.*

Printed in the United States of America
Q-C-C

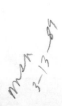

For
Margaret, Jason, Melissa, Chad and Tiffani

PREFACE

THIS laboratory manual and workbook is the outgrowth of several years of struggling to find the most concise, clear and feasible approach to experiential learning about radiographic technique and quality control. It arises out of the philosophy that hands-on experience and active student participation in learning result in much better understanding and retention of the subject matter and ultimately lead to more competent practitioners of radiography.

Many radiography educators agree with this philosophy but find that laboratory time is at a premium when scheduling several students for practical exercises. Experiments must have very explicit directions, they must be concise and to the point, and present analytical questions that are clear to the student and easy for the instructor to score. This manual attempts to meet that need. A comprehensive coverage of practical technique considerations and the quality control methods that relate directly to them is provided in only 25 experiments that can be easily accommodated over two semesters in a typical two-year radiography program.

The manual is student oriented. Instructions include tips for understanding the labs and answering the questions, as well as warnings concerning experimental errors commonly committed by students. Two *practice* laboratories are provided to introdue the students to the proper evaluation of radiographic images. By using these practice labs, the students learn how to properly operate a densitometer, how to obtain quantitative measures of all of the image qualities, and how to avoid confusing one image quality for another.

An effort was also made to build in enough flexibility to each laboratory experiment to accommodate individual program resources and preferences. This was done in two particular ways: First, labs with several possible components such as screen speeds or grid ratios were written to include every feasible variation. Instructors may direct students to those portions of the lab dealing with available components and ignore the remainder. Second, every lab involving a specific radiographic technique also provides blanks for alternate techniques to be written in. Instructors may make any adjustments necessary for their particular equipment limitations without having to *rewrite the book.* Further, a technique adjustments section provides recommendations for compensating techniques according to any combination of generator and screen speed.

Although this manual was designed to be used in conjunction with the *Fuchs's Principles of Radiographic Exposure, Processing and Quality Control* textbook, it is adaptable to any program curriculum. The quality control labs may follow each corresponding technique lab, similar to the organization of the textbook, or they may be separated as a group for use in a quality control course. The two worksheets at the end provide a comprehensive review of the students' ability to synthesize all of the principles of radiographic technique.

It is sincerely hoped that this manual will become a valuable instructional aid for radiography programs which emphasize practical learning.

Q.B.C.

CONTENTS

LABORATORY MANUAL AND WORKBOOK
FOR
**FUCHS'S PRINCIPLES OF RADIOGRAPHIC
EXPOSURE, PROCESSING AND
QUALITY CONTROL, Third Edition**

GENERAL INSTRUCTIONS

Correlation of Laboratory Manual and Textbook

THE Third Edition of *Fuchs's Principles of Radiographic Exposure, Processing and Quality Control* was written for use as a textbook in radiography courses on imaging, technique, processing, equipment monitoring, sensitometric quality control, and those principles of physics *directly* related to these topics. Like this manual, it is organized according to radiographic variables rather than image qualities. Each chapter deals with a specific variable such as mA or kVp and discusses its effects upon each basic image quality. At the end of each radiographic variable chapter, there is a section on quality control for that variable. It lists the specific standards of acceptable deviation for the variable and how to perform QC tests on it.

It is strongly recommended that students be required to thoroughly read the textbook material for a given radiographic variable *before* proceeding to the laboratory experiment on it. In this way, the laboratory experiment will serve as a learning reinforcement mechanism, rather than as an incomplete and usually confusing introduction to the subject.

Most importantly in regard to this laboratory manual, each chapter ends with a concise *summary* of the effects of the variable upon each image quality and guidelines for controlling the variable. When a student experiences confusion over the results of any laboratory experiment or question in this manual, a brief and clear explanation of the relation of that variable to the image quality in question can be found by scanning the corresponding chapter *summary* for italicized key words, which are the image qualities. Such use of the chapter summaries will provide the student with the necessary information to understand the laboratory questions, in most cases. If the student is still confused after reviewing the chapter summary, he/she should then return to the chapter text for a complete discussion of the variable. Care has been taken to ensure that there are no questions in the laboratory experiments which are not addressed in the textbook. This does not mean that the answers are always given outright but that sufficient information is provided that the student should have no trouble synthesizing the answer to a question if the concepts in the text are understood.

Technique Adjustments for Different Machines and Equipment

The techniques suggested in each of the experiments in this manual are selected for a SINGLE-PHASE radiographic unit using HIGH-SPEED CALCIUM-TUNGSTATE INTENSIFYING SCREENS with high-speed film, and automatic developing for 90 seconds at 92-96 degrees Fahrenheit, using Plexiglass™ phantoms.

These techniques should be consistent from one experiment to the next, and within a given experiment. Therefore, if you do not achieve proper densities on the first few experiments, figure out what adjustment is necessary and adjust all of the techniques in the book by the same proportion to get good results.

The following gross adjustments are recommended as a starting point if your machine or equipment does not coincide with the above:

1. FOR THREE-PHASE MACHINE:	Cut mA values or exposure times exactly in half for all labs.
2. FOR PAR-SPEED SCREENS:	Double mA values or exposure times for all experiments.
3. FOR REGULAR RARE-EARTH SCREENS:	Cut mA values or exposure times roughly in half for all labs.
4. FOR THREE-PHASE MACHINE WITH PAR-SPEED SCREENS:	The listed techniques should be close.
5. FOR THREE-PHASE MACHINE WITH REGULAR RARE-EARTH SCREENS:	Cut overall techniques to about $1/4$ those listed for all experiments, using mA and time.
6. FOR OTHER CHANGES:	Refer to the chapters on machine phase and intensifying screens in *Fuchs's Principles of Radiographic Exposure, Processing and Quality Control, Third Edition*.

Further adjustments may be needed for rubber phantoms, different processing variables, mA stations that are out of calibration, etc. Your instructor can help you with these problems.

Blanks are provided on each experiment for alternate techniques to be written in. Once a needed relative change or percentage of change is determined, you should be able to go through the entire manual adjusting all techniques by this amount and writing the results into the alternate technique blanks.

Whatever adjustments are made, be absolutely sure that you do not alter the *relative* changes that are made in the factor under study for a given experiment. For example, if the experiment is on exposure time, and each listed time is double the previous one, be sure that your changed times maintain this doubling relationship, and don't change times at all if the adjustments can be made using mA.

Common Experimental Errors Leading to Poor Results

1. Not *zeroing* the densitometer before measuring. Observe the densitometer reading with no film as you turn the zeroing knob all the way up and down the range. Make sure that you are set to the *middle* zero mark. (A –1.0 will read as zero again.)
2. Step-wedge penetrometers do not produce the realistic amount of scatter radiation which a real patient does, so on some labs the penetrometer measurements will be unrealistically low.
3. On radiographs of body phantoms, it is sometimes difficult to place the densitometer light aperture exactly where you had it on another film, which causes some inaccuracy. Always pick large enough density areas with fairly homogeneous densities, such as a compact bone area or joint space. The trabecular small densities in the mar-

row of a long bone make that a poor spot to measure density.

4. When placing two objects next to each other on a film, don't forget that one may scatter some radiation into the near side of the other. Take your density measurements away from the side that was close to the other object.

5. For an experiment to be valid, *all* other variables, other than the one under study, must be kept equal throughout the experiment. These are too numerous to list, but the most likely problems you will encounter are:

a) mA stations are often out of calibration.

b) Timers are often inaccurate.

c) Processing temperature and concentration (replenishment) vary considerably. When you can, run two films simultaneously or take several exposures on one 14 × 17 inch film.

d) Using different screens or film during the experiment, especially if one is older than the other. When the lab has not been used for several days, it is a good idea to load fresh film in the cassettes that you will use.

e) Changing collimation, distance, or focal spot in the middle of your experiment.

f) Changing machines or phantoms in the middle of your experiment.

6. When taking contrast measurements, be sure to select two film densities that are quite different (one much lighter than the other), so the contrast will be measurable. Always use medium-level densities, not pitch-black or blank areas.

Tips for Answering Laboratory Questions

1. Be sure you observe ONLY those films which the question is asking about; e.g., don't look at "Part B" films when answering "Part A" questions in a lab.

2. Answer only the question at hand. Do not get off on other subjects. Most questions can be answered in one sentence or one word.

3. Read questions carefully and do exactly what they say.

Review: Fundamental Determinants of Radiographic Image Qualities

1. **Density Changes:** Caused by remnant *intensity* (number) of x-ray or light photons reaching the film.

2. **Contrast Changes:** Caused by proportion of *scatter* radiation produced (percentage of Compton interactions) in the patient and reaching the film, or by movement which superimposes different densities.

3. **Noise:** Caused by random scattering of signal (x-ray beam), various artifacts, the creation of false images from movement, and poor resolution of the signal by image receptor systems.

4. **Sharpness of Recorded Detail:** Controlled by *geometry*; specifically by distances, focal spot size, and emulsion crystal sizes and thicknesses.

5. **Magnification:** Controlled by *geometry*; specifically by TFD/TOD ratio.

6. **Distortion of Shape:** Controlled by geometrical *alignment* and *angles* of x-ray tube, part of interest and image receptor (film).

Rounding Numbers and Averaging Results

Round all numbers to the nearest one hundreth (e.g., a calculator reading of 1.518012 should be written down as 1.52).

If you have four change ratios, two from a phantom and two from a step-wedge, you can:

1. Average all four by adding them and dividing them by four, or
2. Average the two phantom measurements. Then average the two step-wedge measurements separately. When answering questions, report both numbers and speculate why one result is different from the other, if it is (see #2 and #3 under the previous section on "Common Experimental Errors Leading to Poor Results").

Significant Change

1. *Density:* A fluctuation in density is not apparent to the human eye until it exceeds a 30 per cent change.

   It is not unusual for mA stations on x-ray machines to be as much as 10-25 per cent off of calibration. Processor temperatures fluctuate up and down, there are fluctuations in electrical supply, and many other factors may vary.

   Due to these many variables affecting density, it is difficult to prove that any change of less than about 15 per cent is in fact due to the experiment itself. To state that an experiment affected density, your numbers should show changes greater than 15 per cent.

2. *Contrast:* A change in contrast should be greater than 0.1 to be considered significant.
3. *Sharpness of Recorded Detail:* Any change is significant.
4. *Magnification/Distortion:* Changes of less than 1 millimeter should be considered insignificant.

Calculating a Range of Insignificant Change for Density

A. Calculate 15 per cent of X (either of your numbers).
B. Subtract this number from X. Record it.
C. Add this number to X. Record it.
D. The insignificant range is from "B" to "C" from the above two numbers.

If a result falls within this range, it is insignificant, and you cannot say that any real change took place as a result of the experiment. If a result falls outside this range, a change definitely took place.

EXAMPLE PROBLEM: Film A Density = 1.88
                 Film B Density = 1.66
                 Film C Density = 2.20

To compare films B and C to film A: 15% of 1.88 = .28
                                     1.88 – 0.28 = 1.60
                                     1.88 + 0.28 = 2.16

The insignificant range is 1.60-2.16; therefore:

Film B is essentially the same density as Film A because 1.66 falls within the range.

Film C is significantly darker than Film A because 2.20 is beyond the range.

Likewise, a change ratio falling between 1.7 and 2.3 may be considered as a doubling.

LABORATORY PRACTICE #1

Determining Density and Contrast Changes

Name _____

PROCEDURE

Expose a knee phantom on two masked-off halves of a 10 × 12 inch high-speed screen cassette on the tabletop using the following techniques. Be sure to label Exposure #1 and Exposure #2 with lead markers. Process your films.

Exposure #1: 200 mA, 1/20 (0.05) sec., 60 kVp
Exposure #2: 200 mA, 1/20 (0.05) sec., 80 kVp

Alternate Techniques:
Exposure #1 _____
Exposure #2 (30% increase in kVp) _____

ANALYSIS

A. *Density:*
   1. Estimate visibly on an illuminator how much darker Exposure #2 is than Exposure #1. Express this as a *factor,* e.g., 1.25 times darker, 1.50 times, 2 times, etc.

   2. Select an area within the *bone* image which has a fairly homogeneous density. This area should not have trabecular lines running through it as in the marrow but should consist of compact homogeneous bone. Where there are many small details of differing densities, the accuracy of your measurements on a densitometer is reduced, because it averages out the detail densities covered by its aperture and it is difficult to place the densitometer aperture *exactly* over the identical spot for each film. Circle this area on both radiographs with a grease pencil or marker and label it *A.*

   Select an area *within* the phantom image which represents a soft-tissue density. A wide portion of an open joint space is a good area for this. This density area must be quite different than the first one in order to obtain good contrast measurements. In this case, it should be considerably darker than the first area found in the bone. Circle this area with a grease pencil or marker and label it *B*.

Check to make sure that the densitometer is *zeroed* properly by taking a measurement without any film in it. If it reads within 0.02 of zero, it is close enough. Take measurements of the circled areas on your radiographs and record them below. Be careful to place the densitometer aperture only over the area of interest, without adjacent, different densities under it.

Exposure #1: Area A density: _____

Area B density: _____

Exposure #2: Area A density: _____

Area B density: _____

3. Compare only the *Area A* densities between Exposure #1 and Exposure #2. Which exposure is densest?

4. Divide (using a calculator, if available) the lesser Area A density number into the greater. The number you get will be the density change ratio (abbreviated ΔD), and represents the factor by which one exposure is darker than the other.

Record this number: ΔD = _____

5. Densitometers measure darkness at the same proportion as the human eye sees it. Compare your ΔD measured with the densitometer to the visual estimate you made in Question #1 above. Are they close? Which one do you trust more?

B. *Contrast:* Contrast is determined by comparing two densities on the same film.
   1. On an illuminator, visibly estimate which exposure has a greater *difference* be-

tween Area A and Area B. Which exposure has higher contrast?

2. Calculate the *contrast* for each film by dividing the smaller density number (Area A) into the larger (Area B) and record it below:

Exposure #1 C: _____

Exposure #2 C: _____

3. Which exposure has higher measured contrast?

4. Does this agree with your answer to Question #1?

5. Calculate the contrast change ratio (ΔC) by dividing the smaller contrast number into the larger. How much *more* contrast does one exposure have than the other?

ΔC = _____ times more contrast.

C. *Sharpness:* Sharpness may be accurately measured on the image of a special resolution pattern device which will be described in a later experiment. For the first several experiments, however, sharpness will be estimated visibly by choosing an edge of bone or other anatomy and observing whether it abruptly stops or gradually fades into the adjacent density. Do NOT confuse contrast with sharpness. An image may look *brighter* against the background density, but the edge may not be any sharper.

Closely examine the same portion of the same edge of bone on Exposure #1 and Exposure #2. Is one sharper than the other? If so, which?

MILLIAMPERE-SECONDS

Laboratory Experiment #1

Name _____

Score_____

PART A

Procedure

Using a step-wedge penetrometer, make a series of four exposures, using the techniques listed below, tabletop with a 14 × 17 inch high-speed screen cassette. Use the same focal spot size for all exposures. The exposure times suggested may have to be adjusted for equipment. Use a new section of film each time, and number your exposures with lead markers.

Fixed = 60 kVp

Exposure #1: 1/30 (0.033) sec., 100 mA
Exposure #2: 1/15 (0.066) sec., 100 mA
Exposure #3: 2/15 (0.13) sec., 100 mA
Exposure #4: 2/15 (0.13) sec., 200 mA

Alternate Techniques
Fixed kVp = _____

Exposure #1 = _____
Exposure #2 = _____
Exposure #3 = _____
Exposure #4 = _____

Analysis

1. Select a specific step of the penetrometer and circle the same area on each exposure. Measure the radiographic density in the selected area for each radiograph with a densitometer. Record these values in the spaces provided below. Calculate the density change ratios (ΔD), by dividing the smaller number into the larger

Exposure #1 density = _____

ΔD = _____

Exposure #2 density = _____

ΔD = _____

Exposure #3 density = _____

ΔD = _____

Exposure #4 density = _____

12

2. Note the density change ratios obtained in No. 1. When exposure time or mA is doubled, how much does the radiographic density change on the average?

3. Are these density changes within plus or minus 15 per cent of what they should be? If not, what things could cause the inaccuracy?

4. Pick two exposures with medium densities and measure on the densitometer the density of a step *adjacent* to the step you measured on the step-wedge penetrometer in Question #1. Calculate the contrast of each film by dividing the smaller step density into the larger:

Exposure A: step A density: _____

                        C = _____

            step B density: _____

Exposure B: step A density: _____

                        C = _____

            step B density: _____

5. Compare the contrast levels measured in No. 4. Do changes in exposure time or mA have a significant (more than 0.1) effect on radiographic contrast?

PART B

Procedure

Using a step-wedge penetrometer, make a series of three exposures using different mA

13

and exposure times which produce the same total mAs, as listed below, tabletop with an 11 × 14 inch high-speed screen cassette. Use the same focal spot size for all exposures. Use a different section of film each time, and number your exposures with lead markers.

Fixed: 56 kVp

Exposure #1: 100 mA at 1/10 (0.1) sec. = 10 mAs
Exposure #2: 200 mA at 1/20 (0.05) sec. = 10 mAs
Exposure #3: 300 mA at 1/30 (0.033) sec. = 10 mAs

Alternate Techniques
Fixed kVp = _____

Exposure #1 = _____
Exposure #2 = _____
Exposure #3 = _____

Analysis

The mAs/density relationship can be examined and evaluated by measuring the radiographic densities of the penetrometer with the aid of a densitometer.

1. Select a specific step of the penetrometer and measure the radiographic density on the same step for each exposure with a densitometer. Record these values in the spaces provided below. Calculate the density change ratios (ΔD), by dividing the smaller numbers into the larger.

Exposure #1 density: _____

ΔD = _____

Exposure #2 density: _____

ΔD = _____

Exposure #3 density: _____

ΔD = _____

Exposure #4 density: _____

2. As long as the total mAs remains the same, should the particular mA and time combination used affect radiographic density?

3. Should the total mAs be directly proportional to radiographic density?

4. Note the density change ratios obtained in No. 1. On the average, was density maintained within 15 per cent by maintaining total mAs in this experiment?

5. Give an example of why it is important to be able to manipulate different mA and exposure time while maintaining total mAs.

PART C

Procedure

Using a phantom pelvis, make four exposures with different mAs values, at about 20 per cent increments, changing time only if possible. Sample techniques are listed below for use with 80 kVp. Use 10 × 12 inch high-speed cassettes in the Bucky mechanism. Number your exposures with lead markers.

Exposure #1: 200 mA at 1/4 (0.25) sec. = 50 mAs
Exposure #2: 200 mA at 3/10 (0.3) sec. = 60 mAs = 20% increase
Exposure #3: 200 mA at 7/20 (0.35) sec. = 70 mAs = 40% increase
Exposure #4: 200 mA at 2/5 (0.4) sec. = 80 mAs = 60% increase

Alternate Techniques

Exposure #1 = _____
Exposure #2 = _____ = 20% increase
Exposure #3 = _____ = 40% increase
Exposure #4 = _____ = 60% increase

Analysis

1. *Visually* evaluate the radiographic images on an illuminator. Be sure to look at the image densities within the phantom rather than the background density. Compare films #2, #3, and #4 with film #1. Which is the *first film* on which the radiographic density of the image is noticeably darker than on film #1? What percentage of mAs increase does this represent?

2. The actual *minimum* percentage change in mAs required to cause a visible change in radiographic density must fall *between* the film which does not show an obvious density difference and the film which does show an obvious difference. Make a rough estimate, then, of the *minimum* percentage by which mA, time, or mAs must be increased when the radiologist asks for a *little darker* film.

3. Convert this minimum percentage into a rounded factor (a rough ratio or fraction) by which mA, time, or mAs must be changed to see a visible film density change.

4. Observe the radiographs visibly on an illuminator. Can you detect any significant difference in the sharpness of image edges caused by mA or exposure time change?

ADEQUATE PENETRATION

Laboratory Experiment #2

Name _____

Score _____

Procedure

Make a series of four exposures of the pelvis phantom using 10 × 12 inch high-speed cassettes in the Bucky mechanism. Number your exposures with lead markers, and use the techniques listed below:

Alternate Techniques

Exposure #1: 50 mAs, 80 kVp   Exposure #1 = _____

Exposure #2: 100 mAs, 40 kVp   Exposure #2 = _____

Exposure #3: 200 mAs, 40 kVp   Exposure #3 = _____

Exposure #4: 400 mAs, 40 kVp   Exposure #4 = _____

Analysis

1. On Exposure #1, has a satisfactory density been achieved?

2. Have satisfactory densities been achieved on Exposures #2, #3, or #4 with their increasing mAs values?

3. Do you believe that a satisfactory density level on the film would be achieved if you increased your mAs to 1000?

4. Can increasing intensity compensate for poor penetration?

5. Reword the principle of radiographic technique in Question No. 4, in terms of *kVp* and *mAs,* that this experiment demonstrates.

KILOVOLTAGE-PEAK

Laboratory Experiment #3

Name _____

Score _____

Procedure

Make two exposures of a step-wedge penetrometer on the tabletop using a 10 × 12 inch high-speed screen cassette masked off into two sections, as listed below, and number each exposure with lead markers.

	Alternate Techniques
Fixed = 5 mAs	Fixed mAs = _____
Exposure #1 = 74 kVp	Exposure #1 = _____
Exposure #2 = 110 kVp	Exposure #2 = _____
(50 per cent increase)	(50 per cent increase)

1. Choose a specific step of the penetrometer and, using a densitometer, measure the radiographic density of this area for each image and record below. Calculate the density change ratio by dividing the smaller number into the larger and record below.

> Exposure #1 density = _____
>
> Exposure #2 density = _____
>
> ΔD = _____

2. Note in No. 1 the effect of increasing the kVp by 50 per cent, and compare this to the effect of increasing the mA by the same percentage. Which of the factors would have a greater influence on radiographic density?

3. Which factor, mAs or kVp, affects density in direct proportion and which affects it in an exponential fashion?

4. Record the densities for Exposures #1 and #2 from Question No. 1 as the *step #1* densities below. For *step #2* measure a step adjacent to the first one. Calculate the contrast on each exposure by dividing the smaller number into the larger.

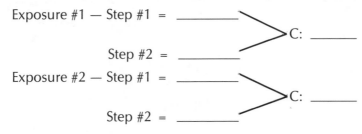

Exposure #1 — Step #1 = _____

Step #2 = _____

C: _____

Exposure #2 — Step #1 = _____

Step #2 = _____

C: _____

5. Compare the contrast obtained at 110 kVp to that obtained at 74 kVp in No. 4. What is the effect of increasing kVp on radiographic contrast: increase, decrease, or no change?

PART B

Procedure

Series #1: Using a phantom elbow, make a series of four exposures tabletop with a high-speed 14 × 17 inch screen cassette masked off into four sections. Use techniques, increasing kVp in steps of 2, as listed below. Be sure to number your exposures with lead markers.

Alternate Techniques

Fixed = 15 mAs	Fixed mAs = _____
Exposure #1: 40 kVp	Exposure #1 = _____
Exposure #2: 42 kVp	Exposure #2 = _____
Exposure #3: 44 kVp	Exposure #3 = _____
Exposure #4: 46 kVp	Exposure #4 = _____

Series #2: Using a phantom skull in PA position, make four exposures using the Bucky mechanism with high-speed 10 × 12 inch cassettes and techniques increasing kVp in steps of 2 as listed below. Be sure to mark your exposures.

Fixed = 30 mAs	Fixed mAs = _____
Exposure #1: 90 kVp	Exposure #1 = _____
Exposure #2: 92 kVp	Exposure #2 = _____
Exposure #3: 94 kVp	Exposure #3 = _____
Exposure #4: 96 kVP	Exposure #4 = _____

Analysis

1. *Visually* observe the radiographs on an illuminator. On the elbow films, which kilovoltage level is the first to demonstrate an *obviously* darker radiographic density from the original exposures? How much of an increase in kVp was this?

   On the skull films, which kilovoltage level is the first to demonstrate an *obviously* darker radiographic density from the original exposure? How much of an increase in kVp was this? Is the kVp change needed for a visible density change the same for all ranges of kVp?

2. Circle a specific homogeneous density area within the radiographic images of the first three of each series of radiographs. Measure the radiographic density with a densitometer and record the value below. Calculate the density change ratios by dividing the smaller number into the larger:

   Series #1
   Exposure #1 — density = _____

   ΔD: _____

   Exposure #2 — density = _____

   ΔD: _____

   Exposure #3 — density = _____

   Series #2
   Exposure #1 — density = _____

   ΔD: _____

   Exposure #2 — density = _____

   ΔD: _____

   Exposure #3 — density = _____

3. For each series, calculate the average density change ratio by adding the two density change ratios above and dividing by two.

Series #1 average density change ratio for 2 kVp: _____

Series #2 average density change ratio for 2 kVp: _____

4. Compare in No. 3 the average density changes produced at 90 kVp to those produced at 40 kVp for 2-kVp increment increases. Do these changes in kVp have equal effects on density in all ranges?

5. Is the use of kVp manipulation for the control of radiographic density as accurate as the use of mAs?

6. When might kVp manipulation be justified (as opposed to mAs manipulation) in controlling film density?

7. What would you say is the *overall* minimum change in kVp required to see a visible change in radiographic density, as a rule of thumb?

8. Visually compare Exposure #1 with Exposure #4 in the first series. Do changes in kVp have an effect on the sharpness of the recorded details?

15 PER CENT RULE FOR kVp

Laboratory Experiment #4

Name _____

Score _____

Procedure

Using 10 × 12 high-speed screen cassettes, make a series of three exposures of the skull phantom in PA position using the Bucky mechanism. Use the same mA station for all exposures, if you can, and label your films. Adjust total mAs and kVp as listed below. The kVp is increased in increments of roughly 15 per cent, while the mAs is cut in half each time.

Alternate Techniques

Exposure #1: 40 mAs at 80 kVp   Exposure #1 = _____

Exposure #2: 20 mAs at 92 kVp   Exposure #2 = _____

Exposure #3: 10 mAs at 106 kVp   Exposure #3 = _____

Analysis

1. Select a small homogeneous medium-density area within the image of each film and circle it. Using a densitometer, measure the density of each point and record it below. Calculate the density change ratios between #1-#2, #1-#3, and #2-#3 by dividing the smaller number into the larger.

Exposure #1 - density = _____

ΔD (1-2) = _____

Exposure #2 - density = _____ ΔD (1-3) = _____

ΔD (2-3) = _____

Exposure #3 - density = _____

2. Note the average density change ratio in No. 1. Are the radiographic images of each film comparable, within 15 per cent, in their overall radiographic density?

Can you see significant visible density differences on a medium-density area?

3. Does the 15 per cent rule for kVp work for density control?

4. What would happen if you used the 15 per cent rule in several steps to reduce kVp too far? (See Lab No. 2)

5. What would happen if you used the 15 per cent rule in several steps to increase kVp too much? (See Lab No. 3)

6. Based on questions #4 and #5, what is the *maximum* number of steps of 15 per cent increase or decrease you would recommend using?

MACHINE PHASE

Laboratory Experiment #5

Name _____

Score _____

Procedure

In a radiology department with both phases of equipment, make three exposures as listed below on a knee or skull phantom, using a high-speed screen in the Bucky tray. Determine a good technique and list it below for a single-phase machine. When changing to a three-phase machine, be sure to use the same collimation, distance, screen speed and focal spot size. Label your films.

Phantom Used: _____

Film #1: Single-Phase Technique: _____ mAs at _____ kVp

Film #2: Three-Phase Technique: _____ mAs at _____ kVp

Film #3: Three-Phase, One-Half mAs: _____ mAs at _____ kVp

Analysis

Select a fairly homogeneous, small area on the phantom image and circle it on each film. Using a densitometer, measure the density on each and record it below. (Note: Film #1 is recorded second in the middle.) Calculate the density change ratio by dividing the Film #1 density into the other two.

Film #2 Density = _____

ΔD = _____

Film #1 Density = _____

ΔD = _____

Film #3 Density = _____

1. Note the change ratio between Film #1 and Film #2. On Film #2, did density increase or decrease when changing from a single-phase to a three-phase machine? By what factor?

2. Note the density change ratio between Film #1 and Film #3. On Film #3, did cutting the mAs to one-half, when changing to a three-phase machine, restore the density to within 15 per cent of the original single-phase density?

25

3. What rule can you make for maintaining radiographic density when changing from single-phase to three-phase machines and vice versa?

4. Can you visually detect a difference in contrast between Film #4 and Film #3? If so, describe it. (You may take actual measurements if you wish.)

—

5. Can you detect any change in sharpness of detail between Film #1 and Film #3.

6. Select two or three procedures from the technique charts for each machine and compare the total technique from the single phase to the total technique from the three phase (using the 15 per cent rule to adjust for kVp differences). Do the charts roughly follow the rule you wrote in Question #3?

COMPENSATING FILTRATION

Group Laboratory Experiment #6

Name _____

Score _____

Procedure

Using a thorax phantom, collimate to expose the AP thoracic spine on a 14 inch or 7 inch film using the technique below. Take a second film with a wedge filter attached to the collimator and an additional 8 kVp to compensate for the filter. Be sure that the thinner end of the wedge filter is toward the abdominal end of the phantom.

Technique = 50 mAs at 76 kVp   Alternate Technique = _____

Analysis

Visually compare the two radiographs on an illuminator. Observe specific areas: (1) T1 to T4 and (2) T10 to T12.

1. Describe the difference between the two radiographs in Area #1 (T1 to T4) regarding density only:

2. Describe the difference, if any, between the two radiographs in Area #2 (T10 to T12) regarding density only:

3. Describe what the second radiograph would appear like, in terms of density, if the wedge filter had been added *without* any increase in technique:

4. Can you visually detect any significant difference between the two radiographs in regard to contrast, sharpness of detail, or distortion?

5. Describe what the second radiograph would appear like, in terms of density, if the wedge filter had been placed with the thick end toward the abdominal portion of the phantom:

FIELD SIZE LIMITATION

Laboratory Experiment #7

Name _____

Score _____

Procedure

Center the lumbar spine of an abdomen phantom on the table in lateral position. (You may need sponges and sandbags or clamps to hold it in place.) Select a technique of 100 mAs and 90 kVp using high-speed screen cassettes. Number your films with lead markers.

Alternate Technique = _____

Film #1 Open the collimator field size to 17 × 17 inches and use a 14 × 17 inch film.

Film #2: Place an extension cylinder or cone on the collimator. (If you do not have one, collimate to a 5 × 5 inch square.) Center over one of the lumber vertebrae. This time use an 8 × 10 inch cassette in the Bucky.

Analysis

1. Select two different, homogeneous density areas on the phantom image. Measure these densities on a densitometer, record them below, and calculate the indicated contrast levels by dividing the smaller number into the greater.

Film #1
density #1 _____
density #2 _____
C: _____

Film #2
density #1 _____
density #2 _____
C: _____

2. Note the #1 *density* for each radiograph. As field size is reduced, does radiographic density increase, decrease or remain equal?

3. Based on the percentage change in density, how much would you estimate the percentage change in mAs is required to restore the density for this much collimation?

4. Why would you not recommend an increase in kVp to compensate for field size limitation?

5. Compare the radiographic contrast measured in Film #1 with that in Film #2. As field size is reduced, does radiographic contrast increase, decrease or remain equal? Explain why.

6. What purpose does a leaded rubber sheet placed on the table just behind the patient's back serve on lateral L-spine radiographs?

GRIDS

Laboratory Experiment #8

Name _____

Score _____

Procedure

Select those grid ratios which are available to you and cross out those listed below that are not available.

Place a 14 × 17 inch high-speed screen cassette on the tabletop, and place various wafer grids on it as listed below with techniques. Place an abdomen/pelvis phantom on top of the grid. Use 40-inch TFD and center carefully to the grid. Be sure to label each film with lead markers.

Determine what ratio your Bucky grid is and fill in the technique change factor by deriving it from the other listed factors.

Fixed = 86 kVp

Film #	Grid Ratio	Technique	Technique Change Factor	Density Measured
1	No grid (standard)	10 mAs	1X	Area A: _____
	Alternate Technique = _____			
2	6:1 grid	20 mAs	2X	Area A: _____
	Alternate Technique = _____			
3	8:1 grid	30 mAs	3X	Area A: _____
	Alternate Technique = _____			
4	10:1 grid	30 mAs	3X	Area A: _____
	Alternate Technique = _____			
5	12:1 grid	40 mAs	4X	Area A: _____
	Alternate Technique = _____			
6	Bucky grid	= _____	_X	Area A: _____
7	15:1 grid	50 mAs	5X	Area A: _____
	Alternate Technique = _____			

Analysis

1. Review the Area A densities. As grid ratio is increased, what would happen to film density (increase, decrease or remain equal) if technique were not adjusted? How does this occur?

2. If the rounded technique change factors above worked, the Area A densities from one film to the next should be within roughly 20 per cent of each other. Is this so? List those which are not.

3. For those you listed in No. 2, estimate what technique change factor you believe would have worked better. List below the technique change factors you would use for each grid ratio. Extrapolate for the grid ratios you did not have available for the experiment.

$$\text{Tabletop non-grid} = 1.0$$

5:1 =	_____
6:1 =	_____
8:1 =	_____
10:1 =	_____
12:1 =	_____
15:1 =	_____
16:1 =	_____

4. On Films #1 and #6, select a different homogeneous density Area B on the phantom image. Take densitometer measurements at these points and record below. Copy the area A measurements from the previous section for these films. Calculate the contrast ratios by dividing the smaller number into the larger number:

Film #1 — Non-grid: Area A: _____

C = _____

Area B: _____

Film #6 — Bucky grid: Area A: _____

C = _____

Area B: _____

5. Note the contrast ratios in No. 4. What is the purpose of adding a grid?

6. How does a grid accomplish this?

7. As grid ratios increase, does contrast increase, decrease or remain equal?

8. Observe the bone edges on the non-grid and the *Bucky* grid exposures. Did use of a grid affect sharpness of detail?

9. Observe a given bone on the non-grid and Bucky grid radiographs. Do grids affect magnification? Do they affect shape distortion?

10. What artifact do you notice on the wafer grid exposures which the Bucky film does not show? Explain how this artifact is eliminated by the Bucky mechanism.

GRID CUTOFF

Laboratory Experiment #9

Name _____

Score _____

Procedure

Without any phantom, expose films with grids as listed below, using 5 mAs at 60 kVp and 40-inch TFD, and a 15:1 focused wafer grid with a 36-42-inch radius. Be sure to label your films with lead markers.

Alternate Grid Ratio = _____

Alternate Technique = _____

Film #1: angle beam 15 degrees *parallel* to (along) grid strips and center.

Film #2: angle beam 15 degrees across grid strips and center.

Film #3: off-center a perpendicular beam across grid strips by 2 inches (mask off unused portion of field).

Film #4: perpendicular, centered beam, but change TFD to 20 inches (cut mAs to $1/4$ original).

Film #5: turn grid upside down with perpendicular, centered beam.

Film #6: change to a 6:1 grid, if available, and angle the beam 15 degrees across the grid strips, as in #2, and center.

Analysis

NOTE: Be sure to observe each film toward the outer edges where grid lines will show the best.

1. List which of the situations above caused grid cutoff only toward one side of the film?

2. Which of the situations above caused grid cutoff equally toward both sides of the film?

3. Compare Films #2 and #6. Does using a different grid ratio affect the severity of grid cutoff caused by angling? If so, which grids are most selective and need more care to

be taken to center and align the CR perfectly?

4. Note Film #1. Does angling *parallel* to grid strips visibly increase grid cutoff?

5. Can you off-center to a grid in a direction parallel to the grid strips?

LABORATORY PRACTICE #2

Measuring Sharpness of Recorded Detail, Magnification, and Distortion

Name _____

Procedure

Place a small bone such as a metacarpal or phalanx and a resolution test template on top of a three- or four-inch sponge and place an 8 × 10-inch high-speed cassette under the sponge. Expose with a light technique as listed below and process the film.

Technique: 100 mA, 1/20 (0.05) sec., 50 kVp

Alternate Technique: _____

Analysis

When comparing levels of sharpness, magnification, or distortion, *any* difference between your numbers should be considered as significant. There is no need to deal with the significant ranges that you use for density and contrast comparisons. (This is because the geometry of x-ray is able to be accurately controlled, whereas electrical characteristics of equipment vary greatly.) Thus, a radiograph showing 1.3 LP/mm has more sharpness than one showing 1.27 LP/mm.

A. *Sharpness of Recorded Detail*

Sharpness of recorded detail may be thought of as how abruptly an edge *stops* and the adjacent density begins. If the edge gradually fades into the adjacent density, then we would say that it is blurred or unsharp and has low recorded detail.

If the edge of two adjacent densities are blurred into each other enough, it becomes impossible to distinguish these two densities as separate objects. Thus, sharpness may be also considered as the ability to distinguish two adjacent details *as separate* details.

The sharper the edges of lines are, the narrower and closer they may be and still be visible as separate lines. So, higher detail means that narrower lines can be recognized. the narrower the lines are, the more of them fit into a given area. For this reason, you can measure recorded detail or sharpness by determining how many lines can be crowded into a given area and still be recognizable as separate lines. The unit of measurement used for recorded detail is *Line Pairs per millimeter,* abbreviated LP/mm.

Refer to your radiograph of a resolution test template. This is a device with a thin sheet of metal foil laminated in plastic. Linear holes are cut in the foil to create alternating light and dark lines on a radiograph when it is exposed to an x-ray beam.

For best results, always place the resolution template *and* any phantoms or bones you are using on a rectangular sponge 2-4 inches thick, with the film under the sponge or in the Bucky, unless the experiment tells you otherwise. When observing a radiograph, scan the line pairs, *from thickest to thinnest,* until you reach the *first point* where you cannot visibly distinguish any more separate lines (they all blur into each other). Find this pair number of the template and read the LP/mm. This is how many line pairs can be distinguished in one millimeter. The higher the LP/mm number, the higher is the sharpness of recorded detail.

Some test templates do not have the LP/mm marked. For this type you must obtain a table from your instructor which lists the LP/mm corresponding to each line-pair number on the template.

(Caution: You may see a second or third area on the pattern image where the lines appear to be clear again. These are areas of false resolution, where two lines have been blurred directly on top of each other. The *first* point where you see the lines blurred into each other is the point where sharpness is lost.)

Based upon the identified blur point of the test template image, record the line pairs per millimeter resolved below:

LP/mm = _____

B. Magnification

Magnification, sometimes called *size* distortion, is the difference in total size between the real object and the image of the object. To determine magnification, measure the object's width and record your measurement; then measure the object's image on the radiograph in *exactly* the same area and record it. Finally, divide the object size into the image size. This will give a *factor* of magnification, which will always be greater than 1.0. For example, a factor of 1.5 means that the image was magnified 1.5 times from the object.

Real bone width = _____

Bone image width = _____

Factor of Magnification = _____

To obtain the percentage of magnification, simply take the number to the *right* of the decimal point in your factor of magnification and multiply it by 100. Record this number below:

Percentage of Magnification = _____ per cent

C. Distortion

Distortion is the difference between the shape of the real object and the shape of the object's image on the radiograph. Distortion may be calculated by first measuring widths and lengths of the object and the image and recording them below; then:

1. divide the width of the *object* into its length. This will give you the ratio of difference between the object's width and its length, an indication of its shape. Record this shape ratio number below.

2. divide the width of the *image* into its length and record this shape ratio below.

3. compare the two numbers you got from #1 and #2. If they are different *at all*, distortion of shape has occurred.

Real object shape ratio = _____ $\dfrac{\text{(length)}}{\text{(width)}}$ = _____

Image shape ratio = _____ $\dfrac{\text{(length)}}{\text{(width)}}$ = _____

Has shape distortion occurred?

NOTE: These procedures explain how to actually measure recorded detail, magnification, and distortion, Many questions on your laboratory experiments may be answered *without* doing these calculations. You can often *visibly* determine:

A. Which resolution pattern image shows the thinnest lines resolved.

B. Which image is magnified most by superimposing the x-ray images on top of each other, and

C. Which image is distorted by observing them side by side or by superimposing them as in B.

INTENSIFYING SCREEN EMISSION

Group Laboratory Experiment #10

Name _____

Score _____

Procedure

Read all of the questions below before proceeding. Open the cassettes listed on the table and observe the light emission during long time exposures (3 or 4 secs.) at the techniques listed below. Watch for color differences and brightness.

$$Exposure \#1 = 50 \text{ mA at } 60 \text{ kVp}$$
$$Exposure \#2 = 50 \text{ mA at } 110 \text{ kVp}$$
$$Exposure \#3 = 10 \text{ mA at } 60 \text{ kVp}$$

Alternate Techniques:

Exposure #1 = _____

Exposure #2 = _____

Exposure #3 = _____

Analysis

1. What color does each screen emit?

   A. Slow detail: _____
      Calcium Tungstate

   B. High-Plus: _____
      Calcium Tungstate

   C. Rare-Earth
      Extremity: _____

   D. Rare Earth: _____

2. Which one glows the brightest?

3. Why does the hi-plus glow brighter than the slow detail?

4. Why would a hi-plus glow brighter than a par?

5. Why does the rare earth glow brighter than the hi-plus?

6. Why must special film be used with most rare-earth screens?

7. As kVp increases, what happens to the brightness of a given screen's emission? Why?

8. What happens to brightness of emission when you decrease the mA station? Why?

9. Why would increasing exposure time *not* increase screen brightness?

INTENSIFYING SCREENS

Laboratory Experiment #11

Name _____

Score _____

PART A: VISIBILITY

Procedure

Select those screen speeds available to you and cross out those listed below which are not available.

Using a par speed 10 × 12-inch cassette and a knee phantom, take an exposure using 10 mAs and 76 kVp at 40 inches TFD. Check to make sure this technique gives you a good medium-density level. Then, if not, adjust all the techniques to do so. Test out the screen speed factors given below by adjusting your technique, exposing and labelling your film as listed below. Use the densitometer to measure density on selected homogeneous areas of the phantom image and record your data below.

Fixed = 76 kVp

Film #	Screen Speed	Technique	Technique Change Factor	Density Measured
1	Par (standard)	10 mAs	1X	Area A: _____
	Alternate Technique = _____			
2	Direct-Exposure	300 mAs	30X	Area A: _____
	Alternate Technique = _____			
3	Slow Detail	40 mAs	4X	Area A: _____
	Alternate Technique = _____			
4	Slow	20 mAs	2X	Area A: _____
	Alternate Technique = _____			
5	High	5 mAs	$1/2$X	Area A: _____
	Alternate Technique = _____			
6	Hi-plus	3.3 mAs	$1/3$X	Area A: _____
	Alternate Technique = _____			
7	Rare-Earth *Regular* with OG Film	2.5 mAs	$1/4$X	Area A: _____
	Alternate Technique = _____			
8	Rare Earth *Medium*	10 mAs	1X	Area A: _____
	Alternate Technique = _____			
9	Rare Earth *Fine*/OG	20 mAs	2X	Area A: _____
	Alternate Technique = _____			

Analysis

1. If the technique factors given worked, each density number on area A should be roughly within 15 per cent of the density (area A) on the standard film #1 (par). List below any that were too far off in your opinion.

2. For those you listed in No. 1, estimate what technique change factor you believe would have worked better. List below for each screen speed the technique change factor you would use when going from a par speed screen to it:

Par = 1.0 _____

Direct Exposure = _____

Slow Detail = _____

Slow = _____

High = _____

High-Plus = _____

Rare Earth (Regular) = _____

Rare Earth (Medium) = _____

Rare Earth (Fine) = _____

3. As receptor speed increases, what happens to film density (increase, decrease, or no change)?

4. Other technique change factors may be derived by placing the factor for the screen you are changing *to* over that which you are changing *from*. Using the technique factors you listed in Question No. 2, calculate technique change factors for the changes listed below:

   Example = From Rare-Earth Regular to Rare-Earth Fine = 2 divided by $1/4$

   = 8X Technique

A. From High speed to Slow Detail   =   _____

B. From High Speed to Direct Exposure   =   _____

C. From High Speed to Rare-Earth Regular   =   _____

D. From Rare-Earth Regular to Rare-Earth Fine   =   _____

E. From Rare-Earth Regular to Direct Exposure   =   _____

5. On Films, #2, #5, and #7, select a different homogeneous density area B on the phantom image. Take densitometer measurements at these points and record below. Copy the area A measurements from the previous section for these films. Calculate the contrast ratios by dividing the smaller number into the larger number:

Film #2 — Direct Exposure: Area A: _____

C   =   _____

Area B: _____

Film #5 — High-Speed Screen: Area A: _____

C   =   _____

Area B: _____

Film #7 — Rare-Earth Regular: Area A: _____

C   =   _____

Area B: _____

6. As receptor speed increases, does image contrast generally increase, decrease, or remain equal?

7. *Exposure latitude* is defined as the margin of error you have in setting technique. The more sensitive a receptor system is to exposure, the less margin for error exists in setting technique. Which of the above combinations allow you the highest exposure latitude?

PART B: DETAIL

Procedure

Place a small dry bone, a coin, and a resolution test pattern on a 2-4-inch sponge and expose using 40-inch TFD tabletop with the techniques listed below.

> Film 1: Cardboard Holder 200 mAs @ 40 kVp
>
> Film 2: High-Speed Screen 3.3 mAs @ 40 kVp
>
> Film 3: Rare-Earth Screen with OG film 1.6 mAs @ 40 kVp

Analysis

1. Determine from each of the resolution template images the LP/mm and record below:

> Cardboard holder _____ LP/mm
>
> High-Speed Screen _____ LP/mm
>
> Rare-Earth Regular Screen _____ LP/mm

2. Note the LP/mm measurements in No. 1. As receptor speed is increased, what happens to the sharpness of recorded detail (increase, decrease or remain equal)?

3. What is the best receptor system to get high sharpness of detail?

   Why must you not use this method on anything other than distal extremities? (Review the factors from Part A.)

4. Can you see a visible change in sharpness of the dry bone images in comparing direct-exposure to high-speed screens?

5. Compare the size and shape of the coin images. Does any magnification or shape distortion occur from different screens?

FOCAL SPOT SIZE

Laboratory Experiment #12

Name _____

Score _____

Procedure

Place a small bone, such as a phalanx, a coin, and a resolution test template side by side on a 6-8-inch rectangular sponge, with one-half of a 10 × 12-inch high-speed screen cassette centered *below* the sponge. Make two exposures at 40 inches TFD using the large and small focal spot factors listed below. Label the exposures and develop.

Fixed: 56 kVp

Exposure #1: 100 mA — small focus at 1/20 (0.05) sec.

Exposure #2: 200 mA — large focus at 1/40 (0.025) sec.

Alternate Techniques:

Fixed kVp: _____

Exposure #1 at small focus: _____

Exposure #2 at large focus: _____

Analysis

1. Observe the radiographic images of the bone, noting the edges of small details. Can you tell visually which image demonstrates the greater sharpness? If so, which?

2. Determine the number of line pairs per millimeter (LP/mm) resolved in each image of the test template and record below:

   Exposure #1 at small focus, LP/mm: _____

   Exposure #2 at large focus, LP/mm: _____

   Which focal spot size resolves greater sharpness?

3. As focal spot size increases, what happens to sharpness of detail (increase, decrease or remain equal)?

4. Ask the instructor for the manufacturer's listed sizes for the two focal spots and list below:

Small F.S.: _____

Large F.S.: _____

Determine the factor by which the large F.S. is bigger than the small F.S. by dividing the smaller into the larger and record:

Focal spot size increase factor: _____

Determine the sharpness change ratio from No. 2 by dividing the small focus LP/mm into the large focus LP/mm and record:

Sharpness change ratio: _____

Now compare the F.S. size change factor to the sharpness change ratio above. Is the relationship between F.S. size and sharpness close to (within 15 per cent) an *inverse* proportion?

5. Measure the length of the real bone and the two bone images and record below; be sure to make all of your measurements in exactly the same part of the bone.

Real bone length: _____

Film A image length: _____

Film B image length: _____

6. Determine the magnification factors for Film A and Film B by dividing the real bone length into each film's image length:

Film A magnification M = _____

Film B magnification M = _____

7. Compare the two magnification factors in No. 6. Would you consider any magnification difference you measured in this lab between the large and small F.S. to be *significant*?

8. Review the textbook diagrams on F.S. size. Do *both* the umbra and the penumbra expand with a larger F.S.? Does this help explain your results? Is focal spot size a controlling factor over magnification of the gross image?

9. Compare the shape of the coin images on the films and the real coin shape. Do changes in focal spot size distort the shape of the images of objects?

10. Compare the bone images. If you maintained equal mAs and kVp, should a focal spot size change have affected density or contrast? If there was a change, what other factors did you change in this experiment which might have caused it?

11. What is a good overall rule of thumb for minimizing unsharpness by using F.S. size?

ANODE HEEL EFFECT

Group Laboratory Experiment #13

Name _____

Score _____

Procedure

Open the collimator to a beam coverage of 4 inches wide and 17 inches long. Place a 14 × 17-inch high-speed screen cassette lengthwise on the tabletop and center the central ray to its middle. Use the technique below and a marker to identify the left side of beam.

Technique = 2.5 mAs at 50 kVp   Alternate Technique = _____

Analysis

1. Place the film on an illuminator. Is there a visible difference in the radiographic density from one end of the exposed strip to the other?

2. Using a densitometer, measure and record the density located 1 inch from the edge of the beam at both ends of the exposed strip. Calculate the *density change ratio* (ΔD), of any difference between the two ends by dividing the smaller number into the larger.

Film #1   density to left _____

_____ = ΔD

density to right _____

3. Locate the position of your tube cathode and anode on the equipment used for this experiment and record it below.

Left side of tube: _____   Right side of tube: _____

4. Is the intensity of the beam less toward the cathod or anode of the tube?

5. Observe the diagrams below. Would a smaller FS increase, decrease, or not affect the

49

anode heel effect?

ANODES

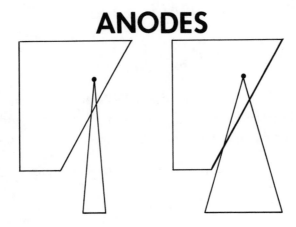

6. Observe the diagrams below showing equal projected focal spot sizes from two different anode bevel angles. Would a steeper target angle increase or decrease the heel effect?

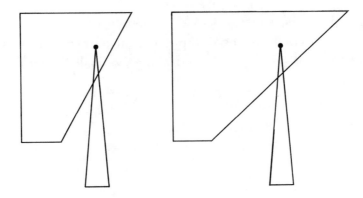

7. In body structures of equal thickness and density throughout their lengths, can the anode heel effect be used to advantage?

8. For a body part that is 5 inches long, can the anode heel effect be used to significant advantage?

9. What positioning rule can you make from this exercise in regard to the anode heel?

TARGET-FILM DISTANCE

Laboratory Experiment #14

Name _____

Score _____

PART A: VISIBILITY

Procedure

Place a step-wedge penetrometer on one-quarter of a 14 × 17-inch high-speed screen cassette, tabletop. Take four exposures using the techniques and the target-film distances listed below and label with lead markers.

Fixed = 56 kVp

Exposure #1: TFD 20'', - 100 mA, 1/30 sec., (3.3 mAs)
Exposure #2: TFD 40'', - 100 mA, 1/30 sec., (3.3 mAs)
Exposure #3: TFD 40'', - 100 mA, 2/15 sec., (13 mAs)
Exposure #4: TFD 30'', - 100 mA, 1/15 sec., (6.6 mAs)

Alternate Techniques:

Fixed kVp = _____

Exposure #1 at 20'' TFD = _____

Exposure #2 at 40'' TFD and same technique = _____

Exposure #3 at 40'' TFD and 4X technique = _____

Exposure #4 at 30'' TFD and 2X technique = _____

Analysis

1. Circle a selected step on the penetrometer for each of the four exposures and measure the radiographic density of each with a densitometer. Record these below:

Exposure #1 — penetrometer _____
step A
density

Exposure #2 — penetrometer _____
step A
density

Exposure #3 — penetrometer _____
step A
density

Exposure #4 — penetrometer _____
step A
density

2. Compare Exposures #1 and #2 in No. 1. What is the effect of increasing TFD on radiographic density if all other factors are kept equal (increase, decrease or no effect)?

3. Why does this density effect occur?

4. Compare the radiographic density of the image produced at 20 inches TFD with the images produced at the other TFD's by calculating the ΔD ratios below.

   A. ΔD ratio of Exposure #1 (20") without changing technique
                    Exposure #2 (40")

      = _____

   B. ΔD ratio of Exposure #1 (20") with technique adjustment
                    Exposure #3 (40")

      = _____

   C. ΔD ratio of Exposure #1 (20") with technique adjustment
                    Exposure #4 (30")

      = _____

5. In No. 4A, how much does doubling the TFD change the density level?

   What is the name of the "law" or principle which this change ratio represents?

6. Based on No. 4B, how much would you estimate should total technique be increased to adequately compensate for doubling your TFD?

7. Based on No. 4C, what technique adjustment would you make for increasing TFD by 1.5 X or 50 per cent?

8. What technique adjustment would you make for *decreasing* TFD to one-half the original?

9. What technique adjustment would you make for decreasing TFD to 3/4 (half-way to 1/2) the original?

10. Copy your *Step A* measurements from No. 1 below. Measure on the densitometer an *adjacent* Step B for only Films #1 and #3 and list below. Calculate the contrast for each exposure by dividing the smaller number into the larger:

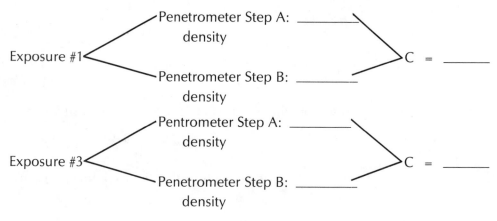

Exposure #1

Penetrometer Step A: _____ density

Penetrometer Step B: _____ density

C = _____

Exposure #3

Pentrometer Step A: _____ density

Penetrometer Step B: _____ density

C = _____

11. Compare the contrast for Exposures #1 and #3 in No. 10. Did a change in TFD have a *significant* (greater than 0.1) effect on image contrast? Can changes in TFD affect the *ratio* of Compton scatter to photoelectric interactions in the patient?

PART B: RECOGNIZABILITY

Procedure

Place a small dry bone, such as a phalanx, a coin, and a resolution test template on a 3- or 4-inch sponge with one-half of a 10 × 12-inch high-speed cassette centered under the sponge. Use the technique and distances listed below. Label your exposures with lead markers.

Alternate Techniques

Fixed = 50 kVp

Exposure #1: 40″ TFD, 5 mAs

Exposure #2: 20″ TFD, 1.25 mAs

Fixed kVp: _____

Exposure #1 at 40″ TFD = _____

Exposure #2 at 20″ TFD = _____

Analysis

1. Observe the radiographic images of the bone. Can you visually see which image demonstrates the better sharpness of detail? If so, which?

2. List the greatest number of LP/mm that you can see clearly defined in each resolution template image.

   _____ LP/mm at 40″ TFD   _____ LP/mm at 20″ TFD

   Which TFD produced the sharpest image?

3. What rule can you make for TFD to produce images with maximum geometric sharpness?

4. Accurately measure the coin's width in mm. Measure the width of each of the recorded coin images. Record these measurements below:

   Real Coin = _____ mm width

   Exposure A (20″ TFD) = _____ mm width

Exposure B (40″ TFD) = _____ mm width

5. Calculate the magnification for Films A and B by dividing the real coin width into each image width and record below. Convert these numbers into percentages of magnification by dividing the whole number into the change (numbers after the decimal) and multiplying by 100:

      Exposure A Magnification = _____ X = _____ per cent
      Exposure B Magnification = _____ X = _____ per cent

6. Compare the magnification factors in No. 5. As the target-film distance is increased, what happens to the recorded size of the image (increase, decrease or no effect)?

7. Considering the results of this experiment, what rule can you make for TFD in reducing magnification?

8. Compare the shape of the coin images on your films and the real coin shape. Do changes in TFD affect shape distortion?

OBJECT-FILM DISTANCE

Laboratory Experiment #15

Name _____

Score _____

PART A: RECOGNIZABILITY

Procedure

Take three exposures tabletop using a coin, a small dry bone (e.g., a metacarpal), and a resolution test pattern. Use an 11 × 14-inch high-speed screen masked off into three sections labelled with lead markers, 40-inch TFD, 2.5 mAs, and 50 kVp, changing only the OFD as listed below:

Alternate Technique = _____

Exposure #1: Place objects directly on the cassette.

Exposure #2: Place your objects on radiolucent sponges to produce an OFD of 4 or 5 inches.

Exposure #3: Place your objects on radiolucent sponges to produce an OFD of 8 or 10 inches; double the OFD on Film #2.

Analysis

1. Observe the radiographic images of the bone. Is there a visible difference in details and sharpness of edges? If so, which is the sharpest?

2. What is the greatest number of LP/mm that you can see clearly defined in each resolution template image?

Exposure #1: _____ Exposure #2: _____ Exposure#3: _____

As object-film distance increases, does geometric sharpness increase, decrease, or not change?

3. Accurately measure the coin's width in mm. Measure the width of each of the recorded images on the radiograph. Record this information below:

Dry bone: _____ mm width

No OFD: _____ mm width

4 inch OFD: _____ mm width

8 10 inch: _____ mm width

4. Using the information provided in Question #3, determine the percentage of magnification in the following problems using the formula provided:

$$\frac{\text{Larger width} - \text{smaller width}}{\text{Smaller width}} \times 100 = M$$

_____ Per cent magnification, no OFD

_____ Per cent magnification, 4-5 inches OFD

_____ Per cent magnification, 8-10 inches OFD

5. As the object-film distance is increased, what happens to the recorded size of the image (increase, decrease or no change)?

6. Is the relationship between OFD and magnification directly proportional (did the size double 100 per cent with double OFD)?

7. Observe the shape of the coin and its images. Does OFD affect shape distortion?

8. Considering the effects of OFD upon both the sharpness of recorded detail and magnification, what general rule can you make for controlling these with OFD?

PART B: VISIBILITY

Procedure

Using two 14 × 17-inch high-speed cassettes tabletop, expose a chest phantom at 40 inches TFD and label each film with lead markers. The exposure factors are 3.3 mAs at 120 kVp. Adjust your OFD as listed below:

      Alternate Technique = _____

      Exposure #1: Phantom directly on film
      Exposure #2: Place phantom on 6-8-inch sponge

Analysis

1. Using a densitometer, measure and record two different homogeneous densities at selected areas in the phantom image for each radiograph below. Calculate the contrast for each exposure by dividing the smaller number into the greater, and record.

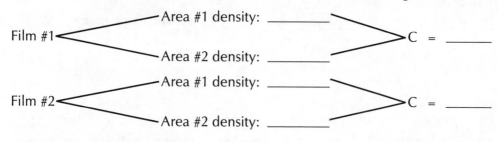

2. Compare the Area #1 densities between Film #1 and Film #2 on No. 1. As OFD is increased, what happens to film density (increase, decrease or no change)?

3. Why does OFD have this effect on density?

4. Compare the contrast ratio for each film in No. 1. Which film has higher contrast? (Remember that the effect measured would be much greater on a very large real patient than it is here on a medium-thickness phantom.)

5. As OFD is increased, what should happen to image contrast (increase, decrease, or no change)?

6. Why does OFD have this effect on contrast?

7. The *air gap technique* employs an increased OFD for very large patients. What is the purpose of this in terms of image quality?

8. Based on your results from Part A, what two problems must be compensated for when using high OFD Air Gap Technique?

9. What factor would you use to partially solve *both* of the problems in question #8?

10. Now, you must compensate for the change made in Question #9 by increasing technique. Would you use mAs or kVp to do this? Why?

TFD/TOD RATIO

Laboratory Experiment #16

Name _____

Score _____

Procedure

Take two exposures of a coin, a small dry bone, and a resolution test pattern, using one-half of a 10 × 12-inch high-speed screen, tabletop, 2.5 mAs and 50 kVp, and distances as listed below. Label each exposure with lead markers.

Alternate Technique = _____

Exposure #1: TFD = 20 inches
OFD = 2 inches
Exposure #2: TFD = 40 inches
OFD = 4 inches

Analysis

1. Magnification can be calculated by dividing the *target-object* distance (TOD) into the TFD. (Don't forget to subtract OFD from TFD to obtain TOD.) Calculate the magnification factor for each film and record:

   Exposure #1 magnification factor: _____

   Exposure #2 magnification factor: _____

2. Compare the two magnification factors in No. 1. What do you notice about these?

3. Measure the size of the two coin images and record below:

   Exposure #1 actual image size = _____

   Exposure #2 actual image size = _____

Is there any difference in magnification?

4. Visually compare the sharpness of detail on the bone images. Are there notable differences?

5. Determine the LP/mm for each film on the resolution test template and record:

           Film #1 LP/mm: _____   Film #2 LP/mm: _____

6. Is there any difference in sharpness of recorded detail?

7. Why did you get the answers you did on these questions?

8. Can TFD or OFD be considered *separately* in controlling sharpness and magnification?

BEAM-PART-FILM ALIGNMENT

Laboratory Experiment #17

Name _____

Score _____

Procedure

Take eight radiographs of a coin and the spherical *head* (not the whole bone) of a dry fe-
mur bone as listed below with various angles and centering. Use 10 mAs and 60 kVp
with high-speed screens tabletop. Place the objects on a 3-inch sponge placed on the
film. Carefully measure and maintain the same TFD, compensating for tube angles, on all
exposures. Mask off small portions to get several exposures on each film. Be sure to number each exposure with lead markers. When off-centering, the CR does not need to be
on the film.

Alternate Technique = _____

Exposure #1: SPHERICAL BONE: beam centered and perpendicular.

Exposure #2: SPHERICAL BONE: beam angled 35 degrees but centered.

Exposure #3: SPHERICAL BONE: beam off-centered 8 inches but perpendicular. (Mask table from unused half of a 16-inch-wide beam with
leaded rubber.)

Exposure #4: COIN: beam centered and perpendicular.

Exposure #5: COIN: beam angled 35 degrees but centered.

Exposure #6: COIN: angled 45 degrees to film. Tape the coin to a 45-degree-
angle sponge at a spot which maintains equal object/film distance (3 inches) as the rectangular sponge provided. Beam
perpendicular to film and centered.

Exposure #7: COIN: angled 45 degrees to film. Tape the coin to a 45-degree-
angle sponge at a spot which maintains equal object/film distance (3 inches) as the rectangular sponge provided. *Beam
perpendicular to coin.*

Exposure #8: COIN: angled 45 degrees to film. Tape the coin to a 45-degree-
angle sponge at a spot which maintains equal object/film distance (3 inches) as the rectangular sponge provided. *Beam
angled isometrically at 22.5 degrees.*

Analysis

Note the direction of tube shift or angle in each case. Remember that the *width* of the
image (perpendicular to the tube shift) must also increase along with its length (parallel
to the tube shift) for *magnification* to be present. You may superimpose images for comparisons.

1. Visually compare Exposures #1 and #2. Does angling the beam cause shape distortion of a spherical object?

2. Did this angle magnify the spherical object (is the width greater too)?

3. Visually compare Exposures #2 and #3. Does off-centering cause the same types of image effects as angling? Why?

4. Compare Exposures #4 and #5. Does angling the beam cause distortion of a *flat object* when the part is parallel to the film?

5. Would off-centering the tube cause shape distortion when the part is parallel to the film? Would it magnify the image?

6. Compare Exposures #4 and #6. Does angling the part in relation to the film cause distortion when the tube is centered and perpendicular to the film? If so, in what way (foreshorten or elongate)? Does it magnify the image (is the width greater, too)?

7. Compare Exposures #4 and #7. Does angling the tube so that it is perpendicular to the

part completely eliminate distortion when the part is angled in relation to the film? Is this image foreshortened, elongated, or not distorted?

8. Compare Exposures #4 and #8. Does angling the tube isometrically adequately eliminate distortion?

9. Are there significant visible changes in sharpness, contrast, or density from changes in alignment, as long as TFD is maintained?

TIMER QUALITY CONTROL TESTS

Laboratory #18

Name _____

Score _____

PART A: SINGLE-PHASE TIMER

Procedure

Take a manual spinning top test on the timer of a single-phase machine for the techniques listed below using two halves of a single 8 × 10-inch cassette. Label your exposures with lead markers. Process the exposed film. Take care not to spin the top so fast that the dots recorded complete a circle and begin to overlap. Use 100 mA and 60 kVp.

Alternate mA and kVp: _____

Exposure #1: 0.07 (1/15) sec.

Exposure #2: 0.15 (1/6) sec.

Alternate Times

Exposure #1: _____

Exposure #2: _____

Analysis

1. Count the number of dots recorded on each exposure and record below. (The dots must be separated but not complete a revolution and overlap each other or the counting may be inaccurate. Such results indicate that the top was spun too fast or too slow.) When counting the dots, include any estimated fractions of a dot. Also, list the number of dots that should be produced at these times:

   Exposure #1 = _____ dots; should get _____ dots.
   Exposure #2 = _____ dots; should get _____ dots.

2. For each exposure, was the actual exposure time exactly accurate, too long or too short?

   Exposure #1: _____

   Exposure #2: _____

3. What is the acceptable limit of accuracy for timers?

4. Do these exposure times fall within the acceptable limit?

                Exposure #1: _____

                Exposure #2: _____

PART B: THREE-PHASE TIMER

Procedure

Take an electrical spinning top test on the timer of a three-phase x-ray machine for the times listed below, at 50 mA and 60 kVp. Any selected alternate times must be less than 1/4 second or the arcs recorded on the film will overlap. Label each exposure with lead markers using two halves of a single 8 × 10-inch cassette. Process the film.

      Alternate mA and kVp: _____

      Exposure #1: 0.1 (1/10) sec.

      Exposure #2: 0.2 (1/5) sec.

      Alternate Times:

      Exposure #1: _____

      Exposure #2: _____

Analysis

1. Pick *one* arc of density recorded on each exposure and carefully measure the degrees of arc with a protractor centered to the axis of the spinning top. List the degrees below: Also list the degrees that should be produced at these exposure times:

      Exposure #1: _____ degrees; should produce _____ degrees.

      Exposure #2: _____ degrees; should produce _____ degrees.

2. For each exposure, was the actual exposure time exactly accurate, too long or too short?

   Exposure #1: _____

   Exposure #2: _____

3. What is the acceptable limit of accuracy for timers? (see textbook)

4. Do these exposure times fall within the acceptable limits?

   Exposure #1: _____

   Exposure #2: _____

MILLIAMPERAGE QUALITY CONTROL TESTS

Laboratory #19

Name _____

Score _____

PART A: LINEARITY

Procedure

Assuming that the timer is accurate, use the following techniques which maintain equal total mAs and kVp to expose a step-wedge penetrometer. For the exposures, mask off four sections of a large cassette and label each exposure with lead markers. Using a single film rather than several eliminates processor fluctuations as a variable in determining density.

>Exposure #1: 50 mA, 1/5 (0.2) sec., 70 kVp
>Exposure #2: 100 mA, 1/10 (0.1) sec., 70 kVp
>Exposure #3: 200 mA, 1/20 (0.05) sec., 70 kVp
>Exposure #4: 400 mA, 1/40 (0.025) sec., 70 kVp
>
>Alternate Techniques maintaining equal total mAs:
>Exposure #1: _____
>Exposure #2: _____
>Exposure #3: _____
>Exposure #4: _____

Analysis

1. Select a medium-density step on the penetrometer images; measure this same step on each exposure with a densitometer and record below:

>Exposure #1 density = _____
>Exposure #2 density = _____
>Exposure #3 density = _____
>Exposure #4 density = _____

2. For each mA station change, calculate the percentage density change by subtracting the smaller number from the larger number and multiplying this difference by 100:

   A) Exp. #1 vs. Exp. #2: _____ — _____ = _____ × 100 = _____%

70

B) Exp. #2 vs. Exp. #3: _____ — _____ = _____ × 100 = _____%
C) Exp. #3 vs. Exp. #4: _____ — _____ = _____ × 100 = _____%

3. What is the acceptable limit of deviation for mA linearity? (See text-book)

4. Do these percentages fall within the acceptable limit?

A) Exposure #1 vs. Exposure #2: _____
B) Exposure #2 vs. Exposure #3: _____
C) Exposure #3 vs. Exposure #4: _____

PART B: REPRODUCIBILITY

Procedure

Take five exposures of a step-wedge penetrometer on a masked-off large film divided into sections using the same technique listed below on all of them.

> Technique: 100 mA, 1/10 (0.1) sec., 70 kVp
>
> Alternate Technique: _____

Analysis

1. Select a medium-density step on the penetrometer images; measure this same step on each exposure with a densitometer and record below:

Exposure #1 density: _____   Exposure #2 density: _____
Exposure #3 density: _____   Exposure #4 density: _____
Exposure #5 density: _____

2. Add up all five densities and divide the sum by 5 to obtain the average density:

Sum density = _____ divided by 5 = Average density: _____

3. What is the acceptable deviation limit for mAs reproducibility? (See textbook)

4. Add and subtract this limit from the average density above to obtain the range of acceptable density deviation:

Acceptable Range: _____

5. Do all of the densities listed in No. 1 fall within this range of acceptance? If not, list those which do not.

KILOVOLTAGE-PEAK AND HALF-VALUE LAYER QUALITY CONTROL TESTS

Laboratory #20

Name _____

Score _____

PART A: WISCONSIN kVp TEST CASSETTE

Procedure

For this lab, instructions supplied with the Wisconsin kVp Test Cassette must be followed to obtain the proper distances and techniques to be used and also to determine the results from graphs which are included. These instructions may be obtained from your instructor.

It is important to use leaded rubber sheets to aid in collimation of the beam over each exposure area of the cassette, so that inaccurate collimators will not result in overlapping exposures. Following the instructions, expose each kVp area marked on the cassette and process the film.

Analysis

For each exposure area, you will find two columns of density dots on the film, one which has equal densities all the way down and one which consists of gradually increasing densities. Visually determine which two or three pairs of dots most closely match in density and measure these on a densitometer. Determine the matching step number. (If one dot is too low and the next is too high in density for an exact match, you should estimate at which fraction of a step a match would occur.)

1. List below the matching step numbers for each test area:

   A) 60-kVp area matching step = _____

   B) 80-kVp area matching step = _____

   C) 100-kVp area matching step = _____

   D) 120-kVp area matching step = _____

   E) HVL matching step . . . . . = _____

2. Refer to the proper graph in the instructions according to the machine phase and kVp used, read off the step number over to the graph line and down to the kVp axis to find the actual kVp, and list these actual kVp levels below:

A) 60-kVp test = _____

B) 80-kVp test = _____

C) 100-kVp test = _____

D) 120-kVp test = _____

E) HVL test = _____

3. What is the acceptable limit of deviation for kVp? (See textbook)

4. Are all of the actual kVp levels listed in No. 2 within this acceptable limit? If not, list those which are not and which direction they are off:

PART B: HALF-VALUE LAYER

Procedure

Pocket dosimeters ranging to 1500 mR with sleeve filters are recommended for this exercise. However, it may be done with any detection device placed under variable slabs of filtration. If pocket dosimeters are used, it is much easier to simply subtract the previous reading from the current reading for each measurement, rather than trying to re-zero or recharge the dosimeter between each measurement. At least three or four measurements should be taken with different thicknesses of filtration. The first reading should be with no filtration added to the beam. Be careful to maintain distances and field size equal on all exposures. Each reading taken will be noted and plotted onto a graph. The last reading taken should be less than one-half of the original reading with no filtration.

Analysis

1. Record below the amounts of filtration added and the reading taken for each exposure. Don't forget to subtract any previous reading on the dosimeter if it has not been re-zeroed.

Exposure #1, no filtration = _____mR

Exposure #2, _____ mm filtration = _____mR

74

Exposure #3, _____ mm filtration = _____mR
Exposure #4, _____ mm filtration = _____mR

2. The first exposure with no filtration will be set as 100 per cent. For the remaining exposures, divide each reading by the Exposure #1 reading and multiply the result by 100 to obtain the percentage of the original exposure produced and record below.

Exposure #2 = _____% of Exposure #1
Exposure #3 = _____% of Exposure #1
Exposure #4 = _____% of Exposure #1

3. On the following sheet of graph paper, plot out these percentages against the amount of filtration in each exposure. Exposure #1 will be plotted at 100 per cent and zero filtration. Draw in a *best fit* line through these plotted dots. (Some variation is natural and the *best fit* line must be found by splitting the difference between some of the plotted dots, in most cases.)

4. On the completed graph, find *50 per cent* of the original exposure, read across to the graphed line and down to the filtration axis. This amount is the half-value layer in aluminum if that is the type of filters used. List the half-value layer below:

HVL at 80 kVp = _____

5. What is the minimum required HVL for operation at 80 kVp? (See textbook)

HALF-VALUE LAYER

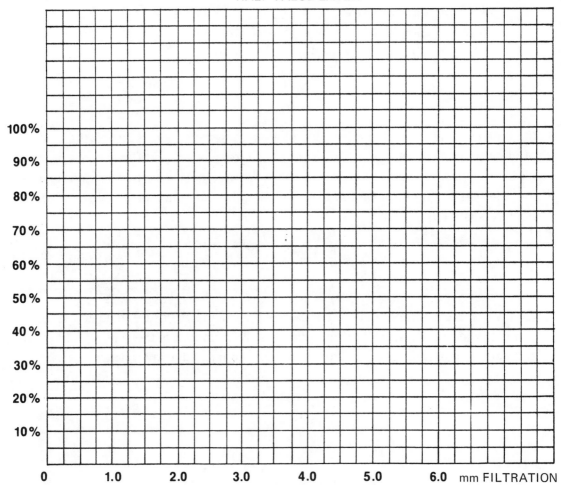

6. Is the HVL measured equal to or greater than that required?

7. If the HVL is not adequate, what does it most likely indicate is needed in regard to adjusting the equipment?

FOCAL SPOT QUALITY CONTROL TESTS

Laboratory #21

Name _____

Score _____

PART A: WISCONSIN TEST TOOL

Procedure

Using the Wisconsin focal spot test tool placed on a direct-exposure holder, set the TFD at 24 inches and expose it with the two different focal spot techniques listed below, masking off two halves of a single film. It is important that you place the tool so that the lines in the groupings run lengthwise and crosswise to the x-ray tube (hence, to the focal spot) and not diagonally. Label each exposure with lead markers. Process the film.

Exposure #1, small focus: 100 mA, 1/10 (0.1) sec., 80 kVp
Exposure #2, large focus: 200 mA, 1/20 (0.05) sec., 80 kVp

Alternate Techniques:
Exposure #1, small focus: _____
Exposure #2, large focus: _____

Analysis

1. Observe the line groupings on an illuminator. The lines run *perpendicular* to the dimension of the focal spot they are measuring. To determine the length of the focal spot, observe the line groups running crosswise. Scan visually from the largest group toward the smallest group until you find the *first* grouping in which the line pairs are not distinct. The grouping *previous* to this one is the smallest grouping resolved. It should demonstrate only three lines per group. Any other number is caused by false resolution (overlapping of double images). Record the number of the smallest grouping resolved below for focal spot length. Repeat the process using the groupings which run lengthwise to obtain the smallest resolved grouping for the crosswise focal spot measurement and record below. Repeat this entire process for Exposure #2 and record below.

Exposure #1, small focus:
Lengthwise dimension, smallest group number = _____
Crosswise dimension, smallest group number = _____

Exposure #2, large focus:
Lengthwise dimension, smallest group number = _____
Crosswise dimension, smallest group number = _____

2. To find the actual sizes of the focal spots, you must obtain a numerical table from your instructor, which is included in the Wisconsin F.S. Test Tool Instructions. The table must be adjusted for a magnification of 4/3 (24 inches TFD over the 18 inches height of the tool). By locating the smallest resolved group in each case on this table, you can read off the focal spot dimension with an accuracy of 16 per cent. Record these measurements below:

Small focus: Length = _____ mm

Width = _____ mm

Large focus: Length = _____ mm

Width = _____ mm

PART B: STAR TEST TEMPLATE

Procedure

Place the star test template at a distance from the film equal to one-half of the TFD. (If using a 14-inch stand provided with the template, place the x-ray target at 28 inches TFD.) It is important to align the pattern so that the Maltese cross formed by the line pairs runs lengthwise and crosswise to the x-ray tube and not diagonally. Take two exposures on a masked-off direct-exposure holder using the techniques below which maintain the same focal spot size but vary mA and adjust kVp. Label the exposures with lead markers and process the film.

Exposure #1: 50 mA, small FS, 1/10 (0.1) sec., 60 kVp
Exposure #2: 200 mA, small FS, 1/10 (0.1) sec., 50 kVp

Alternate Techniques:
Exposure #1: _____
Exposure #2 at increased mA and same FS: _____

Analysis

1. On the resulting star pattern images, scan visually from the periphery inward until you find the *first* point of blur where the line pairs become indistinct. (Apparent areas of sharpness further inward are caused by false resolution when double-images superimpose.) Mark this first blur point on each arm of the star pattern. Measure with a millimeter ruler the diameter between each *pair* of marks across the pattern and record below:

79

Exposure #1, low mA: Lengthwise blur diameter = _____

Crosswise blur diameter = _____

Exposure #2, high mA: Lengthwise blur diameter = _____

Crosswise blur diameter = _____

2. Multiply each of these blur diameter measurements by the factor 0.035 to obtain the actual focal spot dimensions and record below:

Low mA focal spot dimensions = _____ mm X _____ mm

High mA focal spot dimensions = _____ mm X _____ mm

3. If you can, find the manufacturer's listed nominal focal spot size for the small FS on this x-ray tube and list below. Is there a discrepancy between the nominal focal spot size and the actual measured size? If so, why might this be?

4. Compare the focal spot sizes measured at the two different mA values. Is there a difference? Why would increasing mA have an effect upon the effective focal spot size?

BEAM ALIGNMENT AND FIELD SIZE TESTS

Laboratory #22

Name _____

Score _____

Procedure

Place a field size and alignment device over a film cassette, tabletop, or mark off the edges and center of the light field with paper clips or other radiopaque objects. The cassette or exposure holder used must be larger than the field size being checked. If available, also place an x-ray beam vertical alignment test tool in the center of the field test device. The light field must be centered to the screw in the top of the vertical alignment test tool. Be certain to label the field with lead markers denoting which edges are North, South, East and West. Make an exposure with 10 mAs and 60 kVp and process the film.

Analysis

1. Measure the length and width of the actual x-ray field size recorded on the film with a ruler and list below along with the collimator setting for field size:

   Length: Collimator setting = _____ inches; measured = _____ inches
   Width: Collimator setting = _____ inches; measured = _____ inches

2. What is the acceptable limit of deviation for field size accuracy? (See textbook)

3. Are these measurements within the limits of acceptability?

4. For each edge of the x-ray field, measure how far the edge of the black exposed area is from the light field markers and in which direction. List your results below:

   North side = _____ inches off to _____ (direction)

South side = _____ inches off to _____
East side = _____ inches off to _____
West side = _____ inches off to _____

5. Divide each of the deviation measurements from No. 4 by the TFD (40 inches) and multiply this result by 100 to obtain the percentage deviation from the TFD and record below:

North side = _____ % of TFD off
South side = _____ % of TFD off
East side = _____ % of TFD off
West side = _____ % of TFD off

6. What is the limit of acceptable deviation for light field alignment with the actual x-ray field? (See textbook)

7. Which, if any, of the light field edges are out of align by unacceptable amounts?

8. Draw diagonal lines from each pair of corners of *both* the black x-ray field and the demarcated light field in order to locate their respective centers. Measure with a ruler the distance from the x-ray field central ray to the light field central ray and note in which direction it is off and record below:

Light field center is _____ inches off toward _____ from x-ray field center.

9. Divide this measurement by the TFD and multiply the result by 100 to obtain the percentage of deviation from the TFD and record:

Light field center is _____ per cent of TFD off of align.

10. What is the limit of acceptable deviation from the light field center? (See textbook)

11. Is your measurement in No. 9 within this limit of acceptance?

12. Note the image of the screw on the vertical alignment test device. Is the entire screw within the outer edge of the image of the washer? If not, which way is the x-ray beam angled from vertical?

13. How many degrees of deviation from vertical does the outer edge of the washer represent as a minimum acceptable limit? (See textbook)

SENSITOMETRY

Laboratory #23

Name _____

Score _____

Procedure

Expose two different step-wedge images under alternate conditions. Consult with your instructor on which conditions to vary. Some examples include:

A) Exposing two different types of film in a sensitometer or to an x-ray beam using a penetrometer.

B) Exposing two films in a sensitometer or to an x-ray beam with a penetrometer and developing one automatically and one manually.

C) Exposing the same types of film to two extremely different kVp techniques, adjusting mAs to maintain density, using a penetrometer.

Label each exposure with lead markers. When the images are processed, measure and note the densities of every other step on the penetrometer image if it has 21 steps total, or of every step if there are only 11 steps total, beginning with Step #1, #3, #5, etc. Using the graph paper on the following page, plot out the measured densities against the step numbers. Then draw a smooth curve through the plotted points for each exposure. Label these H and D curves for Exposure #1 and Exposure #2.

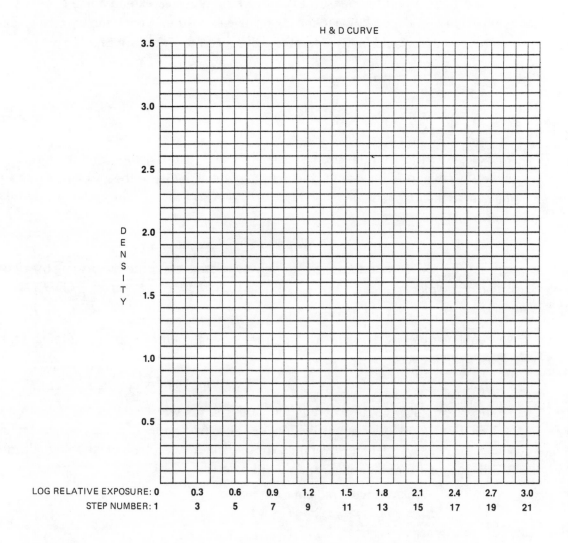

H & D CURVE

LOG RELATIVE EXPOSURE: 0   0.3   0.6   0.9   1.2   1.5   1.8   2.1   2.4   2.7   3.0

STEP NUMBER: 1   3   5   7   9   11   13   15   17   19   21

Analysis

1. Referring to the graph for Exposure #1, what was the density level of the base-plus-fog for this exposure?

2. For Exposure #1, find the density 1.0 *above* base-plus-fog, extend a line over to the graphed curve and then down to the log relative exposure. What is the log relative exposure level that would be used to obtain the speed for Exposure #1?

3. For Exposure #1, obtain the contrast as follows and record below: Find the low density relative exposure by locating the density point at 0.25 *plus* the base-fog, extend a line over to the graphed curve and down to the exposure axis. This is the low density relative exposure.

Low Density Exposure = _____

Repeat this procedure to find the high density relative exposure by locating the density point 2.0 *plus* base-fog.

High Density Exposure = _____

Now subtract the low density exposure from the high density exposure to obtain the exposure difference:

HDE _____ — LDE _____ = Exposure Difference: _____

For the *average gradient* measurement of contrast, the density difference will always be 1.75 (the high density minus the low density). Average gradient is defined as the ratio of the density difference over the exposure difference. To obtain this ratio, divide 1.75 by the exposure difference and record below:

Average Gradient Contrast = _____

4. What difference is there, if any, between the toe portions of the curves for Exposure #1 and Exposure #2? Why would this be so?

5. Which exposure had the fastest speed? Why would this be so?

6. Observing the slope of the body portion of the curves, which exposure produced the highest contrast? Why would this be so?

7. What difference is there, if any, between the shoulder portions of the curves for Exposure #1 and Exposure #2? Why would this be so?

PROCESSING CONTROL CHARTS

Laboratory #24

Name _____

Score _____

Using the processing control charts on the following page, plot and monitor the speed, contrast, base-plus-fog and temperature taken at the same time of day everyday for two weeks or for one month as directed by your instructor. Measurements should be taken during a period of normal load, not first thing in the morning. Draw lines connecting each measurement. Especially watch for continuing trends in the charts and for sudden changes brought on by alterations in the chemistry or processor made on a given day.

Use the measurements taken on the first day as a baseline for comparison and note the appropriate limits above and below this level for acceptable deviation (see textbook). At the end of the period, submit your charts along with a brief report to the instructor describing the causes of any general trends or sudden deviations in the charts.

DATE
DAY M T W T F S S M T W T F S S M T W T F S S

SPEED

CONTRAST

FOG

TEMPERATURE

PERSONAL REPEAT ANALYSIS

Laboratory #25

Name _____

Score _____

Procedure

For a period of two weeks or for one month, as directed by your instructor, save all of your throwaway radiographs regardless of cause and store them in a safe place. Also, keep track of the total number of radiographs you have taken during this period. At the end of the period, count the total number of repeats necessitated and record below.

Total exposures taken = _____   Total repeats taken = _____

1. Divide the total number of exposures you took for the entire period into the number of repeats necessitated and multiply this result by 100 to obtain your repeat percentage rate:

Personal repeat rate = _____

2. What is the national average repeat rate? What is an *ideal* repeat rate for a radiology department, realistically speaking? (see textbook)

3. Sort the repeats into the various categories listed below and record the number of repeats in each area. Divide the total repeats into each of the categories and multiply the result by 100 to obtain the percentage of repeats necessitated in each category:

   A) Positioning Factors = _____ = _____ per cent of total.
   B) Technique Errors = _____ = _____ per cent of total.
   C) Darkroom Errors = _____ = _____ per cent of total.
   D) Patient Motion = _____ = _____ per cent of total.
   E) Other = _____ = _____ per cent of total.

4. Do you personally need the most improvement in positioning, technique control, or patient control?

5. As a practicing radiographer, how will you find opportunities to improve on your weakest areas?

COMPREHENSIVE TECHNIQUE REVIEW

Worksheet #1

Name: _____

Score _____

Directions: For each technique change listed at the left, indicate the effect it will have upon each image quality by placing a plus sign in the box if it increases the image quality, a minus sign if it decreases it, or a zero if it is not a *direct* cause of changes in the image quality. Assume that all factors are maintained equal except the listed change. For example, when the x-ray beam is angled, assume that the TFD is maintained equal through compensating tube-to-tabletop distance.

	Density	Contrast	Sharpness	Magnification	Distortion
Increase mA or Exp. Time					
Increase kVp					
Increase Filtration					
From 1-Phase to 3 - Phase					
Increase Field Size					
Increase Motion					
Increase Patient Size					
Increase Grid Ratio					
Increase Screen Speed					
Increase Size of Focal Spot					
Increase TFD					
Increase OFD					
Misalign or Misangle Beam					

MULTIPLE TECHNIQUE PROBLEMS

Worksheet #2

Name _____

Score _____

1. Which of the following produces the greatest density? _____

	mAs	kVp	TFD	Patient Thickness	Screen Speed	Grid Ratio
A.	400	72	40″	22 cm	High-Plus	12:1
B.	100	94	80″	18 cm	Par	10:1
C.	200	72	40″	26 cm	Direct Exp	None
D.	200	82	40″	22 cm	Sl. Detail	None

2. Which of the following produces the greatest density? _____

3. Which of the following produces the greatest patient dose? _____

	mA	Exp. Time	Phase	kVp	Screen Speed	Grid Ratio	Filter
A.	300	1/5	3ϕ	60	Slow	None	3.5 mm
B.	400	0.6	1ϕ	60	High	12:1	2.5 mm
C.	200	0.6	3ϕ	60	High-Plus	15:1	2.5 mm
D.	600	2/5	1ϕ	52	Rare Earth	None	1.5 mm
E.	300	0.8	1ϕ	70	Par	6:1	2.5 mm

4. Which of the following produces the greatest contrast? _____

5. Which of the following produces the sharpest detail? _____

	mAs	kVp	TFD/TOD Ratio	Focal Spot	Grid Ratio	Screen Speed
A.	50	94	10/1	1.2 mm	6:1	Par
B.	50	72	40/1	1.2 mm	None	Rare Earth
C.	30	80	15/1	0.6 mm	16:1	High-Plus
D.	30	82	40/1	0.6 mm	None	Slow Detail
E.	30	94	10/1	1.2 mm	None	Direct Exposure